MEDICARE

simplified

2020 Edition

What Retirees Need to Know
About Medicare in 100 Pages or Less

MEDICARE

simplified

2020 Edition

What Retirees Need to Know About Medicare in 100 Pages or Less

Ashby Daniels, CFP®

Dedication

To every retiree trying to make sense of a complicated government program supposedly designed to serve the American public.

Disclaimer

Nothing in this book constitutes advice. While stating the obvious, by you reading this book, I cannot assess anything about your personal circumstances, your finances, your goals or objectives. Your situation is unique to you, so any opinions or information contained in this book are just that – opinions or information.

Additionally, while we have made every effort to ensure the accuracy of the information contained herein, we are making no representation or warranty as to the accuracy of the material in this book.

Purchasing this book does not create any client relationship or other advisory or fiduciary relationship with the publisher or author. You, and you alone, are responsible for the financial decisions you make.

Medicare is an extremely complex program. As you can imagine a book of less than 100 or even 1,000 pages could not possibly address every possible scenario. Therefore, you should not use this book to make financial decisions. I highly recommend that you seek professional advice from a qualified individual who is authorized to provide such advice with regard to Medicare and all other areas of your financial life.

Table of Contents

MEDICARE

simplified

2020 Edition

Introduction

In my twelve years as a retirement planner and financial advisor, I have fielded hundreds of questions about Medicare. It is clear that Medicare is complex, but the fundamentals need not be overwhelming.

In the world of Medicare, things are not always as they seem. For instance, Medicare Advantage Plans (we'll get into this) are about the only plans you will see advertised on TV or be encouraged to purchase. This is so much the case that many retirees believe it's the only option available to them. They'll end up in an insurance agent's office or on the phone with the goal of "exploring" plans not realizing there is an entire world of alternative options that are, quite often, less expensive and more comprehensive than the plan being pitched at the moment - all so the salesperson can earn a commission.

I think it's important and relevant to state one important fact up front: I <u>do not</u> sell any insurance whatsoever. I have no underlying motivation in you purchasing one plan over another nor do I have any interest in where you decide to purchase your Medicare plan.

Then, why write this book? There are two primary reasons.

First, according to academic research, approximately 66% of bankruptcies were tied to medical issues[1] – either due to the high costs of care or time out of work. Obviously, for retirees, the high cost of care is a more likely culprit. Given the volume of bankruptcies surrounding medical costs, it is my hope that an educational resource such as the one you hold in your hands may save a few retirees from the brink of bankruptcy.

Secondly, because I am a Financial Advisor who works almost exclusively with retirees, I have heard just about every question under the sun about Medicare.

It seems to me that Medicare is a bit of a black box and retirees aren't sure where to turn for information that is easily accessible. In short, people want and need the information, but they don't want to be overwhelmed by the subject matter. I think it is safe to say that reading a 300-page book on Medicare isn't most people's idea of a good time.

In lieu of boring you to death, I have tried to distill the important points I believe retirees need to know about Medicare into a short, easy-to-understand guide that might even be enjoyable to read.

The unfortunate truth - not that this will surprise you - is that no one is looking out for you and your Medicare decisions. No one is going to ensure that your choices are what's best for you and your family. That responsibility falls 100% on you.

It is also true that many of the choices you make when it comes to Medicare are irrevocable, so it is critical that you make decisions that will be best for you the first time around. Ignorance will never be an acceptable excuse when medical bills come due or when things are not going as you expected.

Your only way to defend yourself against ignorance is unfortunately to educate yourself on this very boring, but important subject.

My hope is that by reading this short guide, you will be prepared to make good decisions for you and your family.

Let's get to it.

Reader's Note: Throughout this book, you will likely encounter terms that are unfamiliar. For that reason, we have included a glossary in the back of the book that includes many of the less familiar terms.

Chapter 1: Medicare & the Problem at Hand

As an advisor working with retirees, the most common question I am asked is, "Should I choose a Medigap policy or a Medicare Advantage plan?"

It's an astute question. But before I answer that question, let's start with the basics.

What is Medicare?

Medicare is a federal health insurance program that covers people who are age 65 or older, certain younger people with disabilities and people with End-Stage Renal Disease. For the purposes of this book, we will only address the 65 and older group.

Generally, when people talk about Medicare, they are talking about Medicare as a comprehensive program, but it is actually broken into parts. The first part is called "Original Medicare" which consists of Parts A and B.

Part A and Part B are designed to cover <u>part</u> of the expenses related to hospital visits and most other medical services. On the surface, based on this statement, it might seem like Part A & B are sufficient to cover your health care costs, but that is highly unlikely. Let me explain.

Gaps in Original Medicare Coverage

There is a gap in the Part A & Part B system coverage. This gap is called coinsurance. If you elect to forego a supplemental policy, you are - whether you realize this or not - taking on part of the financial risk and responsibility for your healthcare costs. In fact, if all you have in retirement is Parts A & B, you will be subjecting yourself to significant (virtually limitless) risk. Let's look at an example.

For example, let's say you recently enrolled in Medicare and opted for just Parts A & B – thereby forgoing any supplemental coverage. Unexpectedly, you are diagnosed with cancer. As you probably know, there are significant costs in front of you such as surgeries that often accompany such a diagnosis, plus the cost of on-going treatments. People on Original Medicare must pay the initial Part A deductible of $1,408 (2020) per benefit period (60 days) plus the Part B deductible of $198. Don't worry about the specific numbers, we will come back to them later in the book.

To be clear, there are additional nuances to the deductible, but beyond the initial responsibility of paying the deductibles, you would be responsible for 20 percent of the cost of most outpatient treatments, doctor visits and the like. And unlike the insurance plan through your employer that you are accustomed to, there is no ceiling on the 20 percent portion you are responsible for!

So, if you were diagnosed with cancer or any other condition, and your bills for the year beyond your deductible are $100,000 (which doesn't take long), you would be responsible for $20,000! You have likely seen medical bills from your healthcare provider and know these costs can quickly add up.

The way you limit this risk is by choosing between two options:

(1) **Medicare Supplement** (also known as and here to forward referred to as Medigap) plus a Part D plan.

(2) **Medicare Advantage Plan** (also known as and here to forward referred to as MA Plans – also called Part C).

Deciding between these two options will be one of the most important Medicare-related decisions you will face. In the case of both Medigap and MA plans, you are guaranteed acceptance into either program regardless of health when you begin Part B of Medicare. Also, in both cases, you will need to pay your Part A (most people get this for free) and Part B premium. To be clear, before you can purchase a MA plan or Medigap plus Part D, you must first have Part A and Part B.

Unlike the employer health coverage you are likely accustomed to, there is no family coverage under Medicare. Your Part B premiums as well as the actual health plans are on a per-person basis. As such, you and your spouse can have entirely separate plans or the same plan and they will be independent of each other regardless of what you decide. You will pay separate premiums and deductibles and could even have entirely different provider networks.

It's also worth noting that not all plans are created equal. You may find yourself paying more (or less) with one company than another for identical benefits.

Unlimited Financial Risk

The gap noted above is how many Americans are – unknowingly – being exposed to virtually unlimited financial risk since there is no annual limit for what you pay out-of-pocket which is where many of the bankruptcies caused by medical expenses stem from.

Therefore, I believe that in most cases, those who can afford additional medical coverage in retirement should purchase it. As we will cover in future chapters, even if you cannot afford additional coverage, there may be some $0 premium options to explore as coverage options. I realize this $0 premium option may sound too good to be true, but this is why I chose to write this book because you cannot take advantage of benefits you don't know about.

Let's review the various pieces of the Medicare program.

Chapter 2: Alphabet Soup – The A, B, Cs (& Ds) of Medicare

What does each part of Medicare cover and how do they all work together? Or do they even work together? Those are good questions. Let's review each part and discuss what each part pays for your health care.

Medicare Part A

Part A is often called "Hospital Insurance" since it covers inpatient hospital care.

Below is a list of services that Part A generally covers:

- **Inpatient Care in a Hospital:** This is care provided after you are formally admitted into a hospital by a doctor. You are only covered for up to 90 days during each benefit period, plus 60 lifetime reserve days.

  o **How will you know you are formally admitted?** You or your caregiver should ask the hospital's medical staff if you are an inpatient or outpatient. Just because you may stay overnight in a hospital does not necessarily mean that you have been admitted. Ask the staff whether you are considered inpatient or outpatient as it will affect what you pay while you are in the hospital as well as what care you may receive after leaving the hospital.

- **Skilled Nursing Facility (SNF) Care:** When receiving care in a SNF, Medicare covers room, board and a variety of other services including administration of medications, tube feedings and wound care. You are only covered for up to 100 days each benefit period if you qualify for coverage. To qualify, you must have spent at least three consecutive days as an admitted patient in a hospital within 30 days of admission to the SNF and you must require skilled nursing or therapy services.

- **Home Health Care:** Medicare covers services in your home if you are homebound and require skilled care. Medicare covers up to 100 days of daily care or an unlimited amount of intermittent care. The requirements to qualify for coverage are similar to SNF care with a slight difference. In order to qualify for home health care, you must have spent at least three consecutive days as an admitted patient in a hospital within 14 days of receiving home health care. (Note: You may also be eligible to receive home health care through Part B if you do not meet the requirements for Part A coverage.)

- **Hospice Care:** Hospice care is often referred to as end-of-life care. This is care you may elect to receive if a provider determines that you are terminally ill. In this case, you are covered for as long as your provider certifies you need care.

- **Select Prescription Drugs:** Part A covers drugs needed during a Medicare-covered stay in a hospital or SNF.

When it comes to Medicare, regardless of the care being provided, it is important to note that Medicare does not typically pay the full cost of your care. You are likely responsible for some portion of the cost-sharing through deductibles, coinsurances and co-payments for all Medicare-covered services.

Medicare Part B

Part B goes by a few names with one being "Supplementary Medical Insurance" abbreviated as SMI. This is <u>not</u> to be confused with Medicare Supplement Insurance (Medigap) that we will cover shortly. More popularly, Part B is often referred to as "Medical Insurance" or "Outpatient Coverage" since it covers many of the day-to-day needs of most retirees.

Part B is split into two primary types of services:

(1) **Services from Doctors and Other Health Care Providers:** These are services or supplies that are needed to diagnose or treat your condition that meet accepted standards of medical practice (and are provided from a licensed health professional who accepts Medicare).

(2) **Preventative Services:** This is healthcare provided to prevent illness or that can be used to detect a condition at an early stage, when treatment is likely to work best. These can be screenings, shots, vaccines, or annual "wellness" visits. You pay nothing for preventative services that are provided by a health care provider who accepts assignment.

Some of the more common services that may be provided under one of the two types of services above are:

- **Ambulance Services:** This is unique and can be hard to define, but for Part B to cover ambulance services in most cases it must be considered true emergency transportation and must be to and from hospitals.

- **Chiropractic Services:** This is only covered when manipulation of the spine is deemed medically necessary to fix a subluxation of the spine – in other words, when one or more of the bones of the spine are out of position.

- **Continuous Positive Airway Pressure (CPAP) Therapy:** Medicare covers a 3-month trial of CPAP therapy if you have been diagnosed with obstructive sleep apnea and may cover you for longer if you meet certain requirements.

- **Durable Medical Equipment:** Examples are walkers, wheelchairs and oxygen tanks.

- **Home Health Services:** These are services covered if you need to receive skilled nursing or therapy care in the home.

- **Limited Outpatient Prescription Drugs:** These are drugs that are administered by your provider or at a dialysis facility.

- **Mental Health Services**

- **Miscellaneous:** Flu shots, Hepatitis B & Pneumococcal vaccines, etc…

- **Screenings:** Cancer, cardiovascular disease, bone density, depression, diabetes, electrocardiogram, HIV, obesity, etc…

- **Therapy Services:** Examples include physical, speech and occupational therapy services provided by a Medicare-certified therapist.

- **X-Rays and Lab Tests**

These are just some of the most common services provided by Part B and this list is by no means exhaustive. Keep in mind, just like with Part A, regardless of the care being provided, it is important to note that Medicare does not typically pay the full cost of your care. You are likely to be responsible for some portion of the cost-sharing through deductibles, coinsurances and copayments for all Medicare-covered services.

Medicare Part C

As noted previously, Part C is also known as the Medicare Advantage Plan program. To learn more about MA plans, please see Chapters 6, 10, 11 and 12.

Medicare Part D

Part D is also known as Prescription Drug Plans. Part D plans are run by private insurance companies that follow specific rules set by Medicare. To learn more about Part D plans, please see Chapter 14.

Chapter 3: Premiums & Deductibles for Parts A & B

Part A Premiums

The cost for Medicare Part A for most people is generally $0 as about 99% of beneficiaries qualify for free Part A. If you or your spouse has worked 40 quarters (10 years) in the U.S., you have already paid for Part A via payroll taxes.

Part A Deductibles

From the Medicare.gov website, for 2020, your Part A deductibles are as follows (the amounts shown are what you are responsible for paying):

Hospital Stay

- $1,408 deductible per benefit period

- $0 coinsurance for the first 60 days of each benefit period

- $352 per day for days 61–90 of each benefit period

- $704 per lifetime reserve day after day 90 of each benefit period (up to a maximum of 60 days over your lifetime)

Skilled Nursing Facility Stay

- $0 for the first 20 days of each benefit period

- $176 coinsurance per day for days 21–100 of each benefit period

- All costs for each day after day 100 of the benefit period

Part B Premiums

Part B premiums are based on your income. The higher costs are due to Medicare's income-related monthly adjustment amount (IRMAA).

The table below shows the premiums due for Part B based on your modified adjusted gross income (MAGI) from two years ago (2018 tax year):

If your yearly income in 2018 (for what you pay in 2020) was			You pay each month (in 2020)
File individual tax return	File joint tax return	File married & separate tax return	
$87,000 or less	$174,000 or less	$87,000 or less	$144.60
above $87,000 up to $109,000	above $174,000 up to $218,000	Not applicable	$202.40
above $109,000 up to $136,000	above $218,000 up to $272,000	Not applicable	$289.20
above $136,000 up to $163,000	above $272,000 up to $326,000	Not applicable	$376.00
above $163,000 and less than $500,000	above $326,000 and less than $750,000	above $87,000 and less than $413,000	$462.70
$500,000 or above	$750,000 and above	$413,000 and above	$491.60

(Table 3.1)

Most people will pay $144.60 per month for their Part B premium. Since there are no "family plans" under Medicare, the premium for a married couple is twice that amount as each spouse must pay their required premium.

For people with limited incomes, they may be eligible for the "Medicare Savings Programs" of which there are four potential programs. These programs can provide financial assistance to pay premiums, deductibles, coinsurance and copayments. If this is of interest, utilize the resources provided in Chapter 20 for more info.

If you are already receiving Social Security or Railroad Retirement benefits, your Part B premiums will be automatically deducted from your benefit payment. If you are not yet receiving the above benefits there are a variety of ways to pay, but the most popular is to sign up for Medicare Easy Pay. Medicare Easy Pay is a free service you can use to have your Medicare premiums deducted from your savings or checking account each month rather than being billed. For more information on Medicare Easy Pay, visit Medicare.gov and search for "Easy Pay."

Part B Deductibles

You will pay $198 for your part B deductible. Once your deductible is met, you are responsible for 20% of Medicare-approved amounts for most doctor services, outpatient therapy and medical equipment – unless of course you have a Medigap plan or MA plan.

Chapter 4: Enrolling in Medicare

When Do You Need to Enroll?

There are multiple opportunities to properly enroll in the Medicare program. Choosing the proper window depends on your personal circumstances. The three primary opportunities are the Initial Enrollment Period, the Special Enrollment Period and the General Enrollment Period.

If you are already receiving Social Security benefits, you will automatically be enrolled for Part A and B upon reaching age 65. You should receive a package in the mail three months prior to your coverage starting with your new Medicare card. The package will also include a letter explaining how Medicare works and informing you that you were automatically enrolled in both Parts A & B.

Let's review the three enrollment opportunities.

Enroll During Your Initial Enrollment Period

Your Initial Enrollment Period is a seven-month window surrounding the month of your 65th birthday. It includes the three months prior to your birth month, your birth month, and three months following your birth month. For example, if you were born in July, your enrollment period would be from April to October the year you turn 65.

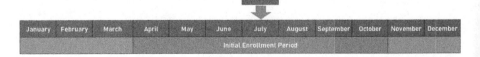

Note: If your birthday falls on the first of the month, your Initial Enrollment Period is the seven months surrounding the month prior to your birth month.

Enroll During a Special Enrollment Period

If you are still actively working and covered by an employer-sponsored health plan, Medicare provides an alternative to your Initial Enrollment Period called a Special Enrollment Period. This is an eight-month period that begins with the month your group health coverage ends or the month your employment ends, **whichever comes first.**

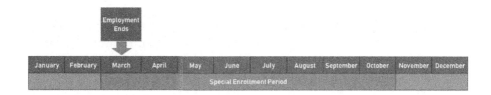

If you are beyond age 65 and still working, it may be worth considering and evaluating whether you should enroll in Medicare Parts A & B, and the plan of your choice (Medigap & Part D *or* MA plan) and dropping your employer health coverage. It is possible that the coverage is better utilizing Medicare and may potentially cost less than your traditional employer plan. You should verify with your employer that you can discontinue your coverage once you are enrolled in Medicare. In many cases, employers are happy to take your family off their health insurance roll. Please note, however, if your spouse is not yet 65 or you have minor children, continuing with your employer plan may be best.

IMPORTANT EXCEPTION: If your retirement or loss of employer provided health coverage ends during your Initial Enrollment Period, then the Special Enrollment Period does not apply. If this is the case, you will need to enroll during your Initial Enrollment Period.

Also Note: COBRA (Consolidated Omnibus Budget Reconciliation Act) coverage, retiree health plans, VA coverage and individual health coverage are not considered creditable coverage by Medicare. To qualify for a Special Enrollment Period, the coverage must be obtained through active employment with an employer with greater than 20 employees. If your company has less than 20 people, you must enroll in Medicare or you may be penalized. See Chapter 5 for additional details.

Enroll During a General Enrollment Period

If you miss your Initial Enrollment Period and your Special Enrollment Period, you may be subject to penalties, but there is still one more opportunity to enroll. The final option to enroll in Medicare is the General Enrollment Period (GEP). The GEP runs from January 1 through March 31 each year with coverage starting July 1.

What if You Have Missed the Enrollment Windows?

Option #1: If you or your spouse is still actively employed and has the option to be covered under their health plan, re-enroll into the health plan during your open enrollment periods. Then, upon retiring, you may make yourself re-eligible for the Special Enrollment Period.*

Option #2: If option #1 doesn't work for you, there may be an additional opportunity for recourse via employment; though it could be tough to pull off. You could go back into the workforce for a company that will offer coverage under their employer health plan – it must be a company with 20 or more employees. Upon retiring this time, you may utilize a new Special Enrollment Period* to sign up for Medicare penalty-free.

However, in either scenario, if you went without creditable health insurance at any point between age 65 and when you eventually enroll for Medicare, you may still be subject to a delayed enrollment penalty. This would be situationally dependent. There is still one more option that may help.

*Note: Not to be confusing, but you only receive one Special Enrollment Period. So, if you missed the entire eight-month window, you will need to utilize Option #3.

Option #3: Appeal. While the U.S. government pretty strictly enforces its rules, there may be opportunities to appeal the penalty if you were given bad information or if they have incorrect data. In most cases, the letter you will receive from the Social Security Administration includes instructions on how to appeal Medicare's ruling. You must have your ducks in a row when appealing the penalty though as they will not accept a plea of ignorance.

Reminder: If you are already receiving Social Security benefits, you will automatically be enrolled for Part A and B upon reaching age 65.

Medigap Enrollment Periods

You may have thought that the enrollment periods just discussed were all you had to worry about. But you would be wrong because Medicare is tricky like that.

Medigap actually has its own six-month enrollment period that begins the month you are 65 or older and enrolled in Medicare Part B. Thankfully, during this six-month Medigap enrollment period, Medigap companies are required to sell you a policy at the best available rate regardless of your health status and they cannot deny you coverage due to preexisting conditions. This is known as guaranteed access rights.

The best available rate, however, is contingent on a few factors such as your age, gender, where you live, your marital status, and whether you smoke (in some states), but you cannot be denied coverage if you enroll during the guarantee issue period.

If you try to buy a Medigap policy outside of protected enrollment periods, companies can refuse to sell you a policy or impose certain medical requirements. If they do agree to sell you a policy, they may charge a higher premium and you may be subject to a six-month waiting period before the Medigap policy will cover pre-existing conditions.

Once you are "IN" your policy is considered guaranteed renewable meaning you will retain the same terms as when you purchased the policy for as long as you keep up with your premiums.

Medicare Effective Coverage Dates

The date your Medicare coverage begins is slightly different than when you sign up so it's imperative upon signing up that you confirm the actual coverage start date. Here's a table showing the probable coverage start dates:

If you sign up for Medicare Part A and/or Medicare Part B in this month:	Your coverage starts:
3, 2, or 1 month before you turn 65	The first day of your birthday month
The month you turn 65	1 month after you sign up
1 month after you turn 65	2 months after you sign up
2 months after you turn 65	3 months after you sign up
3 months after you turn 65	3 months after you sign up
During the Jan 1-March 31 General enrollment period	July 1

(Table 4.1)

Be careful. If you cancel your existing coverage as soon as you sign up for Medicare thinking you are covered, you may be in for a shocking surprise if you visit a doctor in the interim. It is very important to ensure your current health coverage continues until your effective coverage date for Medicare.

Note: If you enroll in Medicare during a Special Enrollment Period, your effective coverage will begin the first month after you enroll. To avoid a gap in coverage using the Special Enrollment Period, enroll in Medicare the month before your employer coverage will end.

How Do You Enroll in Medicare Parts A & B?

Medicare makes the process of enrolling quite easy. You can sign up for Part A and/or Part B benefits in the following ways:

• Online at www.ssa.gov

• By calling Social Security at 1-800-772-1213 Monday-Friday, from 7 AM – 7 PM. TTY users should call 1-800-325-0778.

• Visit your local Social Security office to enroll in person.

• As previously noted, if you are already receiving Social Security benefits, you should be automatically enrolled in Parts A and B. It's always smart to confirm this with the Social Security Administration when you turn 65.

As a best practice, it is often best to protect yourself as you try to enroll in Medicare. Due to the significant penalties (see Chapter 5) that can be incurred for late filing, it is best to record the following as you are enrolling:

• If you apply online, print and save your confirmation page.

• If you apply via phone, record the names of any representatives you speak with including the dates and times in which you spoke with them.

• If you apply in person, ask for a written receipt.

Chapter 5: The Medicare Penalty that Lasts a Lifetime

If you fail to enroll in Medicare during the correct window, Medicare will penalize you. Most people seem to be aware that there is a penalty for late enrollment into the Medicare program. Unfortunately, however, most people are unaware of how significant the penalty is. It is one of the steepest penalties that the federal government imposes on retirees. Perhaps second only to the 50% penalty for failing to withdraw Required Minimum Distributions.

Making matters worse, the Medicare penalty is not a one-time penalty. **It is a penalty you will pay for the rest of your life!** That's a tough pill to swallow to say the least. Enrolling during the proper window can be critical to your long-term financial health.

In this chapter, we will cover what the late enrollment penalty is, and two common reasons retirees fail to enroll on time.

How Much is the Medicare Penalty for Late-Enrollment?

The Medicare late-enrollment penalty is a 10% penalty for every 12-month period you were eligible for Medicare Part B but failed to enroll. So, if you're 70 and didn't enroll in Medicare Part B, there could be a 50% (5 x 10%) penalty.

For example: The starting point for Part B premiums in 2020 is $144.60 per person. If you enroll at age 70 after missing the enrollment periods, your expected premium would be approximately $216.90 per month. This premium figure includes the penalty of about $72.30 per month. This monthly penalty will last the rest of your life!

In lump sum terms based on the above example, if you live to age 85, you could pay over $13,000 in penalties alone. Even if you are just one year late, the cumulative penalties could exceed $3,000.

If your spouse is the same age and hadn't enrolled either, these penalties would be doubled. It gets worse. The penalty estimates noted are not even including the Medicare premium increases that would occur along the way. Pretty steep penalty, right?

And that is just the Part B penalty. Part D also charges its own late enrollment penalty of 1% per month or 12% per year for every year an individual was eligible to enroll but did not. This is getting expensive. More on the Part D late-enrollment penalty in Chapter 14.

Two Common Culprits:

Culprit #1: The most common cause I hear from folks paying this lifelong penalty surrounds the confusion of retiree medical coverage provided by their employer since some companies offer their retiring employees retiree health coverage. In this case, many retirees mistakenly assume this qualifies as employer health coverage for Medicare purposes – and thereby qualifies them for the Special Enrollment Period (see Chapter 4) at the retiree's choosing. It does not.

There are two qualifying factors to be classified as creditable coverage for a future Special Enrollment Period.

- You or your spouse (if covered by your spouse's health plan) must be <u>actively</u> employed.

- You must be receiving health benefits through the spouse that is actively employed.

If that doesn't fit your description, you need to enroll in Medicare.

Culprit #2: If you work for a small employer with fewer than 20 employees, you should get Medicare when you turn age 65. This is because when you turn age 65, your group plan will stop being the

21

primary payer on insurance claims as Medicare assumes the role of primary payer. Your employer plan at that point becomes the secondary payer.

And what happens when you don't have primary coverage because you haven't enrolled in Medicare? You guessed it, surprise bills and possibly a penalty that lasts a lifetime. Luckily, most healthcare providers of employers of less than 20 employees will notify workers turning 65. But this does not always happen the way it should, so it pays to be aware of this caveat to the Special Enrollment Period.

A few additional notes: If you are actively working and over the age of 65, you may prefer Medicare in lieu of your current employer plan for some reason. The most common reason is to have a larger or different network of doctors to choose from.

Something to be aware of if this describes you: If you have family members who are not already covered by or eligible for Medicare and they rely on your employer health coverage, you should likely continue on your employer plan (as long as you are actively employed) until they are Medicare eligible or on their own healthcare.

Now, let's get to the question that I am asked more than any other: "Should I choose Medigap or a MA plan?"

Chapter 6: Medigap vs Medicare Advantage Plans

As we discussed in Chapter 1, to avoid the 20% coinsurance responsibility that comes with Original Medicare, you need to sign up for either a Medigap plan (plus a Part D plan) or a MA plan. These two solutions are two very distinct offerings. Over the next few chapters, I'll highlight the differences and try to identify the types of people for whom each plan might suit best. But first, let's talk about the two types of plans in general terms.

Medigap Plans

Medigap plans are offered by private insurance companies and cover most or all of Original Medicare's out-of-pocket expenses including the 20% coinsurance. Once Original Medicare has paid your claims, the shortfall is then sent to your Medigap plan which will pay its portion of the bill which is typically 100 percent of the shortfall including all deductibles, copayments, and coinsurance if you have the most comprehensive plan.

Medigap has standardized plans in 47 states with Massachusetts, Minnesota, and Wisconsin offering their own plans.

Medigap plans typically come with higher premiums than MA plans, but have few, if any, out-of-pocket expenses. In other words, a Medigap plan may end up costing less despite the higher premium.

The plans are categorized by letter – A, B, C*, D, F*, G, K, L, M, and N. Each plan with the same letter offers the same benefits regardless of state.

*As of 2020, Plans C and F are no longer open to newly eligible enrollees. More info on this in Chapter 9.

Medicare Advantage Plans

These plans are very similar to a typical employer-sponsored health care plan in that they have an accompanying deductible. Additionally, services such as doctor visits, lab work, surgeries and other services are covered by a small co-pay. Each plan places a yearly limit on your total out-of-pocket expenses. Depending on the area that you live, these plans may come in the form of an HMO or PPO and require the use of their network of physicians. An HMO (as many MA plans are) requires seeing a primary care physician as a gatekeeper prior to seeking the help of a specialist. A PPO allows you go out of network at your discretion, albeit with additional costs.

MA plans often include prescription drug coverage, but you will want to verify that any specific drugs you currently take are covered by your specific plan.

Since MA plans are often referred to as Part C plans, another easy way to think of MA plans is the following equation:

Part A + Part B + Part D = Part C

It works this way because MA plans form a contract with Medicare, thus becoming your primary insurance. Most MA plans replace the Original Medicare 80%/20% coinsurance structure with a fixed copayment structure when services are rendered.

MEDIGAP PLANS

Chapter 7: Positives & Negatives of Medigap Plans

Positives of Medigap Plans

• There are no geographic restrictions as you can receive care anywhere that Medicare is accepted (almost everywhere). As a result, you can go to any doctor in the country who accepts Medicare. Medigap will help cover the remaining Medicare out-of-pocket expenses.

> o Author Note: The fact that you can have access to the best doctors in town (or even across the country) may be the most valuable feature of Medigap plans. As we age, the care we receive and the ability to receive it on our terms may offer great comfort in times of stress that typically accompany significant medical issues.

• In most cases, you do not need a referral to see a specialist.

• Less paperwork. Medigap will work on your behalf to send a payment to the doctor or facility without your involvement.

• Several Medigap plans offer emergency medical coverage when traveling out of the country. Please note that you will want to verify with your plan provider what the restrictions are if you intend to travel internationally.

• You can transfer to a MA plan anytime during any Annual Election Period.

- Typically, Medigap policies have lower out-of-pocket expenses than MA plans.

- All plans are standardized by law, so each Medigap of the same letter will cover the same benefits regardless of the insurance company selling it. Please note, however, that these companies can charge different prices for the same coverage, so it pays to shop around.

- Additionally, because Medigap plans are standardized by law, you don't have to worry about what's changing in the plan from year to year, so these plans do not require an annual review like MA plans do.

- Medigap does not provide prescription drug coverage, so you will need to purchase a Part D plan if you wish to receive those benefits. The reason this could be construed as an advantage is because it provides you the flexibility to independently choose from any of the Part D plans to allow you to tailor-fit *your* plan to *your* needs. See below for why this could be considered a disadvantage.

Negatives of Medigap Plans

- Medigap does not provide prescription drug coverage, so you will need to purchase a Part D plan if you wish to receive those benefits. So, if you simply want an all-in-one solution, this is not it. This will require some research to ensure you have a plan that suits your needs. See above for why this could be considered an advantage.

- Does not cover dental care or vision care.

- Premiums are generally higher than that of MA plans.

The Importance of Part D

This section may seem out of place in a chapter on the positives and negatives of Medigap, but I want to be sure that an important point is not glossed over here. That is the critical importance of purchasing a Part D plan if you want to limit your financial risk associated with prescription drugs.

Given drug prices in our country, a Part D plan will be the only protection you have against the skyrocketing prices of one-time and recurring medications. In my opinion, it seems likely that drug prices will continue to increase and a Part D plan is what will protect you from the outrageous prices.

Chapter 8: Who Might Consider a Medigap Plan?

The truth is only you can decide what plan works best for you, but this is food for thought as to who might consider a Medigap plan:

• You are willing to potentially pay a little more in premiums to reduce your overall health care risks meaning you want a more contained cost of healthcare. Because of the way that Medigap plans are structured, your primary expense is the premium since as a general rule, Medicare will pick up 80% and Medigap will pick up the other 20%. The only cost you are generally left with is the Part D premium and copays for prescription drugs via your part D plan.

• You have significant assets.

• You have health concerns or ongoing medical issues. The premiums may be higher, but your out-of-pocket expenses will likely be lower. So, if you are someone with significant medical expenses, the higher premium Medigap policies can end up being a better deal.

• You want the ability to choose which doctor to see, regardless of network or geographic region.

• You like the fact that you do not need a referral to see a specialist.

• You intend to travel domestically or internationally throughout your retirement or you intend to snowbird for part of the year. If this is the case, you will likely derive more benefit from a Medigap plan. This is because under Medigap, you can see any doctor in the country who accepts Medicare, regardless of network, which means you can see almost any doctor in the country. By contrast, if you have a MA plan, any time you are away from your primary care area, each doctor visit will be an out-of-network visit, and therefore cost much more.

Chapter 9: Types of Medigap Plans

Medigap Plan Required Benefits

All Medigap plans must offer the following benefits:

- Hospital coinsurance coverage.

- 365 additional days of hospital coverage.

- Full or partial coverage for the 20% coinsurance for provider and Part B services.

- Full or partial coverage for the first three pints of blood needed each year (if applicable).

- Hospice coinsurance for drugs and respite care.

Medigap Letter Plans

As stated previously, Medigap plans are indicated by a Letter which is why they are known as letter plans.

Because each Medigap policy is required to follow federal and state laws designed to protect you, each letter plan is standardized. This means that all policies of the same letter provide identical benefits regardless of the insurer chosen or the premium charged.

For example, all A plans provide the same benefits as all other A plans regardless of the insurer chosen. This might lead you to choose the insurer offering the lowest premium, but of course we'd be missing the theme of this book. It's never quite that easy.

In essence, once you have settled on the letter plan that works best for you, you can forget thinking about what benefits are provided by whom and focus on the rating of the insurer and their history of premium increases.

Because insurers are incentivized in a few ways to provide good service, a solid rating can be a relatively reliable indication of what you can expect once you enroll in their plan.

New regulations for 2020 have caused some changes to Medigap plans sold to new enrollees. The primary change being that Medigap is no longer allowed to cover the Part B deductible, effectively eliminating Plans C and F (including the Plan F high-deductible option) for new enrollees. If you are already covered by Plan C or F, you can retain your plan as is. And if you were eligible for Medicare before January 1, 2020, but have not yet enrolled, you may still be able to purchase one of those plans.

Note to readers in Massachusetts, Minnesota or Wisconsin: Medigap plans are standardized in a different way in each state. Search for Medigap in "your state" to get more information on those.

Medicare.gov offers a handy chart to help you compare Medigap plans that I include on the following page.

To understand the chart, here are the guidelines:

Yes = the plan covers 100% of the benefit
No = the plan does not cover that benefit
% = the plan covers that percentage of the benefit
N/A = not applicable

Another way of looking at this:
More Yeses = More Comprehensive Coverage

That said, to make this as simple as possible: If you are a new enrollee and are seeking the most comprehensive coverage, the letter plan most likely to fit your desires is Plan G.

Medigap Benefits	Medigap Plans									
	A	B	C	D	F*	G	K	L	M	N
Part A coinsurance and hospital costs up to an additional 365 days after Medicare benefits are used up	Yes	Yes	Yes	Yes	Yes	Yes	Yes	Yes	Yes	Yes
Part B coinsurance or copayment	Yes	Yes	Yes	Yes	Yes	Yes	50%	75%	Yes	Yes***
Blood (first 3 pints)	Yes	Yes	Yes	Yes	Yes	Yes	50%	75%	Yes	Yes
Part A hospice care coinsurance or copayment	Yes	Yes	Yes	Yes	Yes	Yes	50%	75%	Yes	Yes
Skilled nursing facility care coinsurance	No	No	Yes	Yes	Yes	Yes	50%	75%	Yes	Yes
Part A deductible	No	Yes	Yes	Yes	Yes	Yes	50%	75%	50%	Yes
Part B deductible	No	No	Yes	No	Yes	No	No	No	No	No
Part B excess charge	No	No	No	No	Yes	Yes	No	No	No	No
Foreign travel exchange (up to plan limits)	No	No	80%	80%	80%	80%	No	No	80%	80%
Out-of-pocket limit**	N/A	N/A	N/A	N/A	N/A	N/A	$5,560 in 2019 ($5,880 in 2020)	$2,780 in 2019 ($2,940 in 2020)	N/A	N/A

Credit: Medicare.gov

34

Here are Medicare.gov's footnotes for the asterisks from the table:

*Plan F also offers a high-deductible plan. If you choose this option, this means you must pay for Medicare-covered costs up to the deductible amount of $2,340 in 2020 before your Medigap plan pays anything.

**After you meet your out-of-pocket yearly limit and your yearly Part B deductible, the Medigap plan pays 100% of covered services for the rest of the calendar year.

***Plan N pays 100% of the Part B coinsurance, except for a copayment of up to $20 for some office visits and up to a $50 copayment for emergency room visits that don't result in inpatient admission.

MEDICARE ADVANTAGE PLANS

Chapter 10: Positives & Negatives of Medicare Advantage Plans

Positives of Medicare Advantage Plans

• MA plans have the familiar feeling of an employer-sponsored health plan in a lot of ways. (I fully acknowledge that this may be a negative for some people.) It is familiar in the sense that you will have deductibles, co-pays, drug coverage, and physician networks just like most employer plans.

• Many plans include prescription drug coverage. So, if you want an all-in-one solution, this may be a fit. You should verify that the plan you are considering covers your current prescription drugs before enrolling. See below for why this could be considered a disadvantage.

• Commonly covers dental and vision care. Generally, this coverage is for routine annual visits only.

• MA plans may also offer wellness programs (like gym memberships).

• Some MA plans have a $0 premium.**

Negatives of Medicare Advantage Plans

• The downside of having a prescription drug coverage as part of your MA plan is that their formulary could change from year to year, meaning that prescriptions that were previously covered may not be covered in the next year. This will be something to check each and every year. See above for why this could be considered an advantage.

• MA plans can change year by year – they can change approved provider networks, which drugs are covered, number of covered doctors, premiums and out-of-pocket costs. Due to this fact, it would be wise to conduct an annual plan review to ensure it is still the best plan for you.

• Increased costs for going out-of-network as benefits are typically provided in-network. This can be both a geographical and "best doctor" limitation. For example, if you live in an area with multiple health systems, you will likely be limited to the doctors in your network rather than wherever the "best doctor" practices. This "best doctor" drawback can be a real blow to you or your family member if and when a true health emergency arises.

• Generally, you cannot transfer to Medigap plans at will once outside of the guaranteed access period. Beyond that point, you must answer health questions to qualify, at which point you could be denied.

• Benefits are more restrictive than Medigap plans.

• You may need a referral to see a specialist. Because these plans are considered "managed care", providers aim to keep their healthcare costs within budget by trying to prevent overuse. One way providers manage care is by requiring prior authorization from a primary care physician "gatekeeper" for various medical requests.

**Where is the Fine Print?

With regard to $0 premium and ultra-low premium plans, it seems relevant to note, though you will never hear about this from the Medicare Advantage providers, that these providers contract with the federal government and are paid a fixed amount per person (a significant sum that is close to impossible to find) to provide Medicare benefits. According to Philip Moeller, author of Get What's Yours for Medicare, the amount paid by the federal government to a MA plan insurer is approximately $10,000 per enrollee. Insurers also get extra bonuses of more government cheese (cumulatively several billion each year) based on quality ratings. In other words, plans that are rated 4 or 5 stars get extra cash from the government.[2]This is how Medicare Advantage providers are able to offer $0 premium plans and still make a tidy profit along the way.

The incentives seem slightly misaligned here in the opinion of your humble author. How might this work in the real world? If a provider of a MA plan ends up spending less caring for you than the flat fee it receives from the government, it makes more money. This can at least partially explain the desire for outpatient when inpatient may be better or a reluctance to run more tests when something doesn't feel right to you.

Forgive my skeptical nature when considering this issue, but now you at least know why you get a thousand pieces of mail and hundreds of phone calls around your 65th birthday – everyone is vying for the government provided cash cow that is the Medicare Advantage program. With this much money available to providers, it's no wonder we are seeing enrollment in MA plans grow at a phenomenal rate to the point that MA plans now make up about a third of the Medicare business.[2]

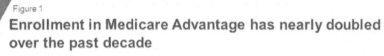

Figure 1

Enrollment in Medicare Advantage has nearly doubled over the past decade

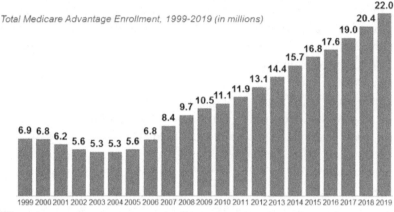

Total Medicare Advantage Enrollment, 1999-2019 (in millions)

	1999	2000	2001	2002	2003	2004	2005	2006	2007	2008	2009	2010	2011	2012	2013	2014	2015	2016	2017	2018	2019
Millions	6.9	6.8	6.2	5.6	5.3	5.3	5.6	6.8	8.4	9.7	10.5	11.1	11.9	13.1	14.4	15.7	16.8	17.6	19.0	20.4	22.0
% of Medicare Beneficiaries	18%	17%	15%	14%	13%	13%	13%	16%	19%	22%	23%	24%	25%	27%	28%	30%	31%	31%	33%	34%	34%

NOTE: Includes cost plans as well as Medicare Advantage plans. About 64 million people are enrolled in Medicare in 2019.
SOURCE: Kaiser Family Foundation analysis of CMS Medicare Advantage Enrollment Files, 2008-2019, and MPR, 1999-2007 enrollment numbers from March of the respective year, with the exception of 2006, which is from April

Figure 1: Enrollment in Medicare Advantage has nearly doubled over the past decade

Credit: kff.org

So, the question becomes, are the incentives to provide care properly aligned with their profit motives? I am honestly not sure. To be clear, this is the case with all insurance. Every little bit extra that is provided technically cuts into their profit margins. But it seems to lack transparency for me which is why I wanted to bring it to your attention.

Another note on the $0 premium plans. We know that no Medicare plan is free as you may still pay deductibles and copays for covered services and you are still responsible for the Part B premium.

I say this not to lament $0 premium MA plans as they serve a very important role in the lives of many American retirees. This great benefit may be of help for folks who may not have the financial resources necessary to purchase any other coverage. In this case, for folks who cannot financially afford any other coverage, enrolling in a $0 premium

MA plan may be a worthy consideration as it may serve as a way to limit your financial risk with no additional premiums required.

Chapter 11: Who might consider a Medicare Advantage Plan?

I will reiterate that only you can decide, so this is just food for thought. Here are some common reasons to consider a MA plan:

- You want an all-in-one solution. Most plans offer drug coverage as part of the plan (you will want to verify your current prescriptions are covered by the plan you choose).

- You feel comfortable with your health plan through work and would like to keep a similar arrangement.

- You like having a primary care physician guide the care you receive.

- You are in particularly good health and are okay with the financial implications if and when that changes. Given the right circumstances, this could amount to quite a savings due to the lower premium MA plan.

- You are not an active traveler domestically or internationally.

Questions to Ask Before Enrolling in a Medicare Advantage Plan

- What is the monthly premium?

- Will the plan cover your preferred doctors and facilities?

- What is the service area for the plan?

- What costs (premiums, deductibles, copayments) should you expect from the plan?

- What is the out-of-pocket maximum for the plan?

- What is the rating of the plan?

- Does the plan cover your monthly Medicare premiums? Some plans will help pay part or all of your Part B premium – this benefit is sometimes called a "Medicare Part B premium reduction."

- How much do you pay for each visit or service (copayments or coinsurance)?

- Do you have any coverage for care received outside of the plan network?

- Do you need a referral from your primary care physician to see a specialist?

- Does the plan cover any services that Original Medicare does not such as dental, vision and hearing?

- Are your prescriptions on the plan's formulary?

- What costs should you expect to pay for your prescription drugs?

Chapter 12: Medigap or Medicare Advantage Plan Premiums

Premiums can vary significantly under both types of plans but typically range between $0 (at times) up to and beyond $300 per month depending on a variety of factors. Some offer discounts for spouses if both enroll. The only way to know what premiums to expect is to get premium quotes from a qualified impartial provider.

It is important to note that in both Medigap and MA plans, higher premiums do not equate to better coverage. Do your research on individual plans to ensure you are getting the most benefits for the premium you are paying. It would also be important to note that these premium costs are not to be considered your all-in costs, as there could be potential deductibles, co-pays, and coinsurance that must be factored in to decide which plan could be a better fit from an overall cost and care perspective.

How Much is a Medigap Plan?

Medigap plan premiums can have a relatively wide range depending on the geographic area and insurer chosen. In Pennsylvania, the approximate premium for a Medigap G plan is around $110 per person. If you are still eligible for an F plan, you may want to verify that the plan premium does not exceed the part G plan by more than the Part B deductible since that is the only difference between the plans.

How Much is a Medicare Advantage Plan?

The average MA plan premium has been declining since 2015 with the average cost per enrollee of $29 per month in 2019.[2] This can vary based on the type of plan selected. There are a lot of plans to choose from – anything from Health Maintenance Organizations (HMO) to Point of Service plans, to Preferred Provider Organizations (PPO) to Private Fee-for-Service plans.

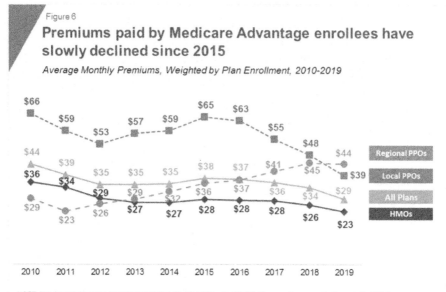

Figure 6

Premiums paid by Medicare Advantage enrollees have slowly declined since 2015

Average Monthly Premiums, Weighted by Plan Enrollment, 2010-2019

NOTE: Includes only Medicare Advantage plans that offer Part D benefits (MA-PDs) because they comprise the majority of Medicare Advantage plans. Excludes SNPs, employer-sponsored group plans, HCPPs, PACE plans, and plans for special populations. The total includes cost plans and PFFS plans (not shown separately), as well as plans with zero premiums. The premiums for a subset of sanctioned plans were not available in 2011, and were excluded from this analysis.
SOURCE: Kaiser Family Foundation analysis of CMS Medicare Advantage Landscape and Enrollment Files, 2010-2019

KFF

Figure 6: Premiums paid by Medicare Advantage enrollees have slowly declined since 2015

Credit: kff.org

There are far more factors to consider than just the premium when choosing a MA plan.

Three tips to consider when deciding which MA plan to purchase:

- Be certain that your doctors and preferred health care providers are approved providers in the plan.

- Be certain your prescription drugs are covered.

- I would favor plans rated 4 and 5 stars.

MA plans can be a great fit for many people. At the very least, these plans put a cap on your maximum annual health expenses. The highest out-of-pocket maximum allowed by any MA plan is $6,700. With healthcare service costs continuing to skyrocket, it's smart to limit your financial risk.

Chapter 13: Changing Plans

What if you change your mind? Can you change plans if you decide an alternative plan is better suited for you?

If you already have Medicare, there is an Annual Election Period (a.k.a Open Enrollment Period) each year when you can select new/different MA plans and drug plans. This period runs every year from October 15 through December 7.

If you are a Medigap participant and decide that Medigap isn't for you, you can always choose to enroll in a MA plan during an Annual Election Period.

But, as you may have guessed, there is a catch if you initially enroll in a MA plan and want a Medigap plan. People who enroll in a MA plan when they are first eligible for Part A at age 65 get a "trial period" of up to 12 months that can allow you to try out a MA plan for one year. If you decide during that time that you prefer a Medigap plan, you can enroll with guaranteed issue rights.

But, if after the first year you want to switch from a MA plan and to a Medigap plan, you would have to answer health questions to enroll in a Medigap plan, in which case you could be denied.

Even switching Medigap plans can be worrisome. There are limited situations where guaranteed issue rights will be in place to switch plans once you have enrolled in Medigap. This is why your decision of which Medigap policy you initially choose is so important.

If you find yourself trying to decide between Medigap and MA plans though, remember that changing FROM Medigap TO a Medicare Advantage plan is much easier than the other way around. This makes the Medigap offering that much more appealing.

Can You Have Both a Medigap AND Medicare Advantage Plan?

No, you cannot. Medigap plans do not work with MA plans. If you have a MA plan, it is illegal for anyone to sell you a Medigap policy unless you are switching back to Original Medicare.

If you join a MA plan for the first time and are unhappy with the plan, you may have special rights under federal law to purchase a Medigap policy and Part D plan if you return to Original Medicare **within 12 months** of joining the MA plan.

Chapter 14: Part D Plans

If you have settled on a MA plan for your health care solution in retirement, you may be able to skip this chapter as most MA plans include prescription drug coverage. Be sure to confirm this though before passing on a Part D plan.

If you have chosen a Medigap plan, you will need prescription drug coverage. Part D provides prescription drug coverage and helps pay for prescription drugs you use at home, plus insulin supplies and some vaccines. These prescription drugs are covered regardless of whether you fill them one time or on a recurring basis. Each plan offered (regardless of insurance company) through Medicare Part D must provide at least a standard level of coverage established by Medicare. Most plans exceed this standard level though.

Each individual Part D plan publishes the list of prescription drugs they cover. This drug list is called a formulary. Each formulary must include at least two drugs in the most prescribed categories, classes and tiers.

Below is an example of how the "tier" system may work:

- Tier 1 – Lowest copayment and includes most generic prescription drugs.

- Tier 2 – Medium copayment and includes preferred, brand-name drugs.

- Tier 3 – Higher copayment and includes non-preferred, brand-name drugs.

- Specialty Tier – Highest copayment and includes very high cost prescription drugs.

All drug plans are different, so you will want to see what drugs are included in which tier based on your needs before settling on a drug plan.

A formulary for one plan may not include the specific drug you may need, but another plan may cover it. So, it's important to check the specific formulary for plans you are considering to ensure your drugs are covered.

It is possible that a plan can make changes to its formulary during the year as drug therapies change, new drugs are released, or new medical information becomes available. If your drug is removed from the list, the insurance provider must do one of two things:

- The plan must give you written notice at least 30 days before the date the change becomes effective.

- At the time of your refill request, they must provide written notice of the change and at least a month's supply under the same plan rules as before the change.

If that is not satisfactory to you and your prescribing physician believes none of the alternative drugs will work for your condition, you can ask for an exception. This may not be as easy as it sounds, but exceptions are often approved through the end of the coverage period at which point you may search for a different Part D plan.

If the exception is not granted and you continue to use a drug that is not on your plan's formulary, you may have to pay full price instead of a copayment or coinsurance

Part D Deductible

Part D deductibles are costs you must pay each year for your prescription drugs before your drug plan pays its share. These deductibles vary based on the drug plan of your choosing, but there are guidelines set by Medicare. For 2020, no Medicare drug plan may have a deductible more than $435. Some drug plans have no deductible, but they cannot exceed $435.

What Should You Expect to Pay for a Part D Plan?

Part D premiums are priced on a per plan basis so what you will pay depends entirely on the plan you choose. The nationwide average in 2020 is about $33 per month. But wait, there's more.

As you might expect, Medicare wants to be sure they are getting their cut if you "make too much money." Below, you will find a table from the Medicare.gov site that shows the Income-Related Monthly Adjustment Amounts. Just like your Part B IRMAA premium adjustment, this is based on your modified adjusted gross income from two years prior. For 2020, your IRMAA charge is based on your 2018 modified adjusted gross income.

If your filing status and yearly income in 2018 was			
File individual tax return	File joint tax return	File married & separate tax return	You pay each month (in 2020)
$87,000 or less	$174,000 or less	$87,000 or less	your plan premium
above $87,000 up to $109,000	above $174,000 up to $218,000	not applicable	$12.20 + your plan premium
above $109,000 up to $136,000	above $218,000 up to $272,000	not applicable	$31.50 + your plan premium
above $136,000 up to $163,000	above $272,000 up to $326,000	not applicable	$50.70 + your plan premium
above $163,000 and less than $500,000	above $326,000 and less than $750,000	above $87,000 and less than $413,000	$70.00 + your plan premium
$500,000 or above	$750,000 and above	$413,000 and above	$76.40 + your plan premium

Table 14.1 - Credit: Medicare.gov

Late Enrollment Penalty for Part D

For those who have settled on a Medigap plan, a common refrain I have heard from lucky folks who do not take any prescription drugs is to skip the Part D plan entirely to save premium cost. The truth of the matter is that you are likely to need some prescription drugs at some point in your future – we just don't know when.

As you might imagine, the Medicare system works best when everyone is involved, both healthy and non-healthy people, since it works on a law of large numbers basis. To "encourage" healthy people to obtain a Part D plan, they charge a late enrollment penalty for Part D just as they penalize late-enrollees into standard Medicare though it is calculated differently.

The Part D penalty is steep. Medicare charges a late-enrollment penalty of 1% per month for every month you are without credible coverage. So, even if you aren't currently taking any prescribed medications, you will likely want to enroll in a Part D plan anyhow. Let's go through how this penalty works.

The 1% (monthly) penalty is based on the national base beneficiary premium (NBBP), which for 2020 is $32.74. Let's say you enrolled into your chosen Part D plan 24 months late. How can we calculate the penalty?

0.24 (24 months x 1% penalty) **x $32.74** (2020 NBBP) **= $7.86**

$7.86 rounded to the nearest $0.10 = **$7.90 monthly penalty**

This $7.90 is the <u>monthly</u> penalty that will be owed every month for as long as you are enrolled in a prescription drug plan, which is probably the rest of your life. This penalty is added to the premium of your chosen prescription drug plan so there is no avoiding it.

Adding insult to injury, this penalty amount will be recalculated annually as the national base beneficiary premium changes year over year – which in most years increases thereby increasing your monthly penalty.

Closure of the Donut Hole

Whether you are new to Medicare or not, you have probably heard of the Part D donut hole. This was the phase of Part D coverage during which you were responsible for more of the cost of your prescription drugs. Over the past few years, the donut hole has been slowly closing.

Starting in 2020, the donut hole is completely closed, which means you will pay, on average, 25% of the cost of your generic and brand-name drugs. That still sounds expensive. That is where catastrophic coverage comes in.

Beware: Despite the donut hole closure, you may still pay more in the donut hole in many cases because you will be responsible for the full 25% of the cost instead of just the copay you paid during the initial coverage phase.

Catastrophic Coverage

Each Part D plan has catastrophic coverage that differs for each plan and it is a major factor in terms of how insurers market their Part D plans. Catastrophic coverage is a bit of a misnomer though, because if you reach your catastrophic coverage level, this does not mean you get every prescription drug for free from that point forward. It means you will now pay "just" 5% of the cost of the drug from that point forward. In the case of some really expensive medications, this can be pricey. Because this little tidbit isn't overly clear in most of the marketing materials, I don't want you to be caught off-guard.

How to Pay for Part D

You can have the premiums deducted from your Social Security benefit or be billed directly. Contact your drug plan to establish your payment plan.

Finding a Part D Plan That's Right for You

Medicare's Plan Finder can offer significant assistance in identifying a prescription drug plan that may work for you. Using their plan finder, you can enter your prescription drugs and it will sort through the available plans and provide a rough approximate of what a year's worth of your medications will cost you. Since drug plans update their formulary each year, it is best not to assume that you are all set once you purchase your Part D plan. Once you create an account on the Plan Finder site, you should be able to update your prescription drugs each year and run an annual comparison to ensure you are making the best plan choice possible.

> ➤ Medicare Plan Finder: www.medicare.gov/plan-compare/

Chapter 15: What Is NOT Covered by Medicare?

As you have learned, Medicare does not cover everything. Here are a few common items that are not covered by Medicare beyond what has been discussed previously:

- Acupuncture.

- Alternative medicine.

- Care provided outside the United States. (Medigap may cover.)

- Concierge care.

- Cosmetic surgery – generally only covered if needed to improve the function of a malformed part of the body.

- Custodial care.

- Dental care including dentures. (MA plans may cover.)

- Hearing aids and exams for fitting them.

- Long-term care.

- Nursing home care.

- Routine foot care.

- Vision care. (MA plans may cover.)

While it is important to have an idea of what Medicare does not cover, I would not assume that something isn't covered just because it is an item listed above. Certain circumstances, based around medical need or otherwise, may cause Medicare to cover it. Always, always, always verify before assuming that a certain service is not covered. But in just the same way, you should verify that something IS covered before proceeding with a care decision as there can be large dollars at stake without realizing it.

You have the right to ask a doctor or facility if whatever care you are receiving will be covered by your Medicare coverage. The last thing you want is a large, unexpected bill to show up in your mailbox.

> ➢ Helpful Tip: If you are wondering whether a specific procedure or equipment is covered, you can visit the "Is my test, item or service covered?" tool on Medicare's site here:

https://www.medicare.gov/coverage

Chapter 16: Health Savings Accounts & Medicare

Health Savings Accounts (HSA) are for individuals who participate in high-deductible health plans. Funds contributed to a health savings account are not taxed when contributed to the HSA, grow tax-deferred, and are distributed tax-free if the funds are used to pay for qualified medical expenses.

For many individuals who have been in high deductible plans and funding their HSAs to prepare for health expenses in retirement, it is important to know a few things:

(1) As soon as you start receiving any benefits from Medicare, you are no longer eligible to contribute to your HSA. This means if you are 65 or older and receiving Social Security benefits that you are not eligible to contribute to an HSA since you cannot decline Part A while collecting Social Security benefits.

(2) If you are enrolling in Medicare during your Initial Enrollment Period (see Chapter 5), you can continue to contribute to your HSA until your effective date of Medicare coverage. For instance, if your 65th birthday is May 8 and you enroll immediately, you can contribute to your HSA from January through April.

(3) If you are enrolling in Medicare outside of your Initial Enrollment Period (see Chapter 5), you must stop contributing to your HSA at least six months before you enroll in Medicare. This is because when you enroll in Medicare Part A, you can receive up to six months of retroactive coverage, not going further back than your initial month of eligibility. If you do not stop your HSA

contributions at least six months prior to Medicare enrollment, there may be tax penalties.

(4) A commonly overlooked topic when it comes to HSAs is including a beneficiary designation. Since this account is not typically considered a retirement asset, many people fail to name a beneficiary which will cause the account to be liquidated and become part of your estate, thereby eliminating the attractive tax benefits that are so popular with HSA accounts. If passed along properly, the HSA will pass to your beneficiary with balances and tax advantages intact.

A couple of additional notes about HSAs. If you find that you are no longer eligible to contribute to an HSA, it does not mean you cannot have an HSA. You can still enjoy the other benefits of the HSA account such as continued tax-deferred growth and tax-free qualified distributions even if you are unable to contribute.

If your spouse is otherwise HSA-eligible, they can still make tax-deductible contributions into their HSA up to the family maximum if you remain covered on a family contract.

What Can Your HSA Dollars Pay For?

You can reimburse yourself, your spouse, or your dependents, income tax-free, for all qualified medical out-of-pocket expenses that are not reimbursed by other insurance or other sources. Some examples include:

- Reimbursement for insurance premiums for Parts A, B, D and MA plans.*

  o Note: Medigap premiums are not reimbursable.

- Copayments and coinsurance.

- Dental and vision expenses.

- Insulin and diabetic supplies.

- Over-the-counter drugs and medicine with a prescription (if not covered by your Part D plan.)

Any distributions from your HSA for non-eligible expenses are included in your taxable income just as if it was a distribution from a 401k or Traditional IRA thereby nullifying one of the great benefits of the account, so it is wise to use HSA funds solely for eligible-medical expenses.

*In order to reimburse your own or anyone else's Medicare premiums income tax-free, the owner of the HSA account must be age 65.

Chapter 17: How Your Investments Can Impact Your Premiums

Few retirees are aware that their portfolio can actually have a significant impact on Medicare premiums. Because Part B and Part D premiums are based on modified adjusted gross income from two years prior (the tax year in which you turn 63 if you plan to enroll at 65), planning for Medicare may actually start at age 62 or earlier.

Modified Adjusted Gross Income (MAGI) is a bit of a mystery to most folks because it doesn't show up on your tax return, so you'll have to crunch some numbers to find it.

 MAGI is your household's Adjusted Gross Income (found on your Tax Return Form 1040 – line 8b for 2019) with any tax-exempt interest income plus certain deductions added back in. For most people, MAGI is identical or very close to AGI. The most common deductions that are added back in are:

- Any deductions you took for IRA contributions.

- Half of your self-employment tax.

- Any deductions you took for student loan interest or tuition.

- Passive income or loss.

- Rental losses.

- Interest from EE savings bonds used to pay higher education expenses.

- Excluded foreign income.

- Employer-paid adoption expenses.

- Losses from a publicly traded partnership.

See Table 3.1 in Chapter 3 to see how your MAGI can impact your Medicare Part B premium.

Beyond your traditional incomes, there are two other scenarios where people could unknowingly alter their Part B premiums and that is when recognizing capital gains or completing Roth conversions.

Capital Gains & Roth Conversions

Over the past decade, we have experienced significant market growth which has resulted in substantial unrealized gains in many taxable accounts. If you are nearing retirement and have been considering making some portfolio changes that will cause some of those gains to become taxable, you may want to do that prior to the year in which you turn 63 or at least two years prior to filing for Medicare.

You may also consider realizing some of those gains prior to age 63 if you are intending to use this portfolio for income purposes in retirement. Otherwise, you may run the risk of having higher Medicare premiums as a result since capital gains will increase your MAGI.

This is the same story for folks planning to pass along as many IRA dollars as possible to their heirs who have been taking advantage of IRA conversions. When converting your Traditional IRA to a Roth IRA, this is a dollar-for-dollar increase in your taxable income - assuming an IRA basis of $0. Again, this will cause an increase in your MAGI. Once you are within two years of enrolling in Medicare, your Roth conversion strategies must account for both tax bracket awareness and Medicare IRMAA awareness as well.

I have found that many investors and their advisors just focus on the conversion part and the tax bill to follow without considering the impact it could have on future Medicare premiums.

If either of the two situations fits your scenario, it's important to note that these Medicare hits may be short-term since the two-year lookback is an annual event. This means that each successive year, they will revisit your MAGI to see where you fall for Medicare premiums.

Additionally, as time goes on, your Required Minimum Distributions (now starting at age 72 thanks to the SECURE Act) may have an impact on your Medicare premiums as well. So, if you are someone who may not need your IRA distributions for retirement income purposes, you may consider taking advantage of the Roth IRA conversion strategy just discussed to reduce your future distributions via conversions in the early years, thereby possibly reducing your Medicare premiums in the process.

As usual, this is all dependent on your financial situation as well as where you fall on the Medicare premium IRMAA table.

Chapter 18: TRICARE for Life & Medicare

Here are a few points worth knowing about the combination of Medicare and TRICARE for Life.

In order to utilize TRICARE for Life, you must be enrolled in Medicare Parts A & B. TRICARE is required to send out a postcard alerting you of this fact prior to TRICARE members turning 65.

Once you are enrolled with Medicare Parts A & B plus TRICARE for Life, Medicare becomes the primary payer of your health costs and TRICARE is secondary. This means all medical claims will first be sent to Medicare with any unpaid amounts sent to TRICARE for Life.

TRICARE for Life also tends to have comparable (and usually cheaper) drug coverage than a Medicare Part D drug plan.

Given the generous benefits that many of our retired servicemembers are to receive from the combination of Medicare Parts A & B and TRICARE for Life, it would be unlikely that you would require any further coverage and you should be rightly skeptical of anyone who says otherwise.

TRICARE members can get assistance enrolling in Medicare at www.TRICARE.mil.

Chapter 19: Planning Around Your 65th Birthday/Retirement

Having a plan of attack for your enrollment in Medicare can keep the process from becoming overwhelming. As such, below you will find a suggested timeline for when you should complete a variety of activities. Regardless of whether you enroll during your Initial Enrollment Period or your Special Enrollment Period, here are some helpful guidelines to follow in the year leading up to Medicare enrollment.

Within One Year of Enrollment

- Get a full physical exam with bloodwork.

- Obtain a copy of your records and medical history for your review.

- Discuss preventative measures and the state of your overall health with your healthcare team.

7-9 Months Before Enrollment

- Verify your eligibility for Medicare benefits by calling 800-772-1213.

- Review current and post-retirement healthcare benefits to determine your overall healthcare options.

4-6 Months Before Enrollment

- Review Medigap Plans with Part D options and MA plan options.

- Inquire with your healthcare team to ensure they accept the coverage you are planning to enroll in.

1-3 Months Before Enrollment

- Enroll in Medicare Parts A & B. (See Chapter 4.)

- Decide between a Medigap/Part D plan and a MA plan.

Chapter 20: Getting Assistance with Medicare

Choosing a plan for your healthcare through retirement is truly a personal choice and can take a bit of time and effort. But the health care you will receive in the future is at stake as are your financial resources, so it is wise to spend whatever time necessary to be sure you get this right the first time. One step you can take to accomplish this is to know your rights.

What Are Your Rights with Medicare?

Medicare is crystal clear about the rights you have as an enrollee in the Medicare program. They are as follows: You have the right to...

- Be treated with dignity and respect at all times.

- Be protected from discrimination.

- Have personal and health information kept private.

- Get information in a format and language you understand from Medicare, health care providers, Medicare plans, and Medicare contractors.

- Have questions about Medicare answered.

- Have access to doctors, other health care providers, specialists, and hospitals for medically necessary services.

- Learn about your treatment choices in clear language that you can understand, and participate in treatment decisions.

- Get Medicare-covered services in an emergency.

- Get a decision about health care payment, coverage of services, or prescription drug coverage.

- Request a review (appeal) of certain decisions about health care payment, coverage of services, or prescription drug coverage.

- File complaints (sometimes called "grievances"), including complaints about the quality of your care.

Now that you know your rights, how can you find qualified help to determine which plan is right for you?

Getting Help Finding a Plan That's Right for You

When choosing between Medigap or MA plans, consider the advantages and disadvantages discussed in previous chapters as well as the costs associated with each. Know the deductibles you should expect, monthly premiums, restrictions on doctors, hospitals, and pharmacies, as well as what your maximum out-of-pocket expenses could be. Educating yourself on the topic of Medicare is not likely to be a pleasurable activity, but a necessary one nonetheless.

There are tremendous resources available where you can obtain personalized assistance to identify which plan to purchase and get just about any question answered you can possibly think of. Below you will find a comprehensive list to accomplish all of that and more. My one encouragement would be to **use these resources**.

You have a right to have your questions answered in a way that you can clearly understand, and you have a right to be treated fairly. You are and always will need to be your biggest advocate. If you are not getting the answers you are seeking, keep trying or utilize an alternative resource from the list that follows.

Medicare Resources

There are several resources available to folks dealing with Medicare that can answer specific questions as they arise. Again, by all means necessary, **use these resources!**

Here are two helpful tips as you begin to search for answers on the below sites: (1) Each site listed contains a "search bar" where you can type in relevant language and you will be directed to pages that may be relevant to your query. (2) You can also search most of these sites by topic. Here are the sites:

- **Medicare.gov website.** The actual Medicare website is a wealth of information. They have an online tool called "What's Covered?" that can tell you whether a specific procedure or piece of equipment is covered. They also have a variety of publications that get into the details about certain aspects of Medicare that you may find useful.

  - ➢ Medicare web address:

    - ▪ https://www.medicare.gov/

  - ➢ Medicare Publications:

    - ▪ https://www.medicare.gov/publications

- **Medicare Rights Center.** This is a national, non-profit consumer service organization that helps ensure access to affordable healthcare. They staff (through paid staff and a significant volunteer force) a national telephone helpline. They can help you understand your benefits, understand how your existing coverage works and even help you find the right coverage for you. They also host an additional website called Medicare Interactive that provides a wealth of information.

  - ➢ Medicare Rights Center web address:

    - ▪ https://www.medicarerights.org/

➢ Medicare Rights Center Phone Number: 800-333-4114

- **State Health Insurance Assistance Program (SHIP).** This federally funded program has thousands of trained volunteers around the country who can help with your Medicare questions and problems. By visiting their site, you can use their "SHIP Locator" to find help closer to home. Once you have found your local provider, there are helplines and other additional websites with important information. The volunteer counselors who answer the helplines can assist you with anything Medicare related including helping you with plan comparison and enrollment, deal with billing problems, and they will even help you file a complaint about medical care or treatment.

    ➢ SHIP web address:

    ▪ https://www.shiptacenter.org/

- **Center for Medicare & Medicaid Services (CMS) website.** CMS is the federal agency that administers the Medicare program.

    ➢ Center for Medicare & Medicaid Services web address:

    ▪ https://www.cms.gov/

- **Social Security website.** Medicare enrollment is handled through the Social Security Administration. Given that fact, it may not be surprising to know that the Social Security website also has some tools to help you find answers to your questions.

    ➢ Social Security web address:

    ▪ https://www.ssa.gov/

- **Healthcare.gov website.** This is the federally facilitated medical marketplace website. It also has tremendous resources regarding just about any question you may have organized by topic.

➤ Marketplace web address:

- https://www.healthcare.gov/

- **Medicare Plan Finder:** Medicare.gov maintains websites to help you sort through the myriad of plans available to you.

  ➤ For MA Plans and Part D Drug Plans:

  - https://www.medicare.gov/plan-compare/

  ➤ For Medigap Plans:

  - https://www.medicare.gov/medigap-supplemental-insurance-plans/

- **Department of Defense:** For information on TRICARE for Life.

  ➤ https://tricare.mil/tfl

- **BOOK: Get What's Yours for Medicare – Maximize Your Coverage, Minimize Your Costs by Philip Moeller.*** In my opinion, this is the most readable book you will find that goes into more of the fine print of Medicare.

*Raymond James is not affiliated with and does not endorse the opinions or services of Philip Moeller.

Epilogue/Conclusion

Throughout this book, I have tried to cover the primary questions and challenges facing today's retirees with regard to healthcare in retirement. As you can imagine though, with thousands of plans across hundreds of networks, it would be impossible for me to discuss each plan or narrow down which plans would be best for you and your family. This is made even more impossible because your situation is unique to you. My sincere hope is that through this book, I have provided the information and resources needed for you to make more informed Medicare decisions.

For more helpful retirement information, please visit my blog at www.retirementfieldguide.com.

I wish you great success in your retirement journey!

Thanks for reading!

-Ashby Daniels

All-Important Disclaimers:

This book is not to be considered advice as I do not know you or your personal situation. I recommend that you work with a Certified Financial Planner professional as you seek to implement any ideas you find herein. Lastly, I am not a tax accountant or an attorney, so please do not take anything stated herein as tax or legal advice in any fashion.

Raymond James Disclaimers: The information contained in this book does not purport to be a complete description of the securities, markets, or developments referred to in this material. The information has been obtained from sources considered to be reliable, but we do not guarantee that the foregoing material is accurate or complete. Any information is not a complete summary or statement of all available data necessary for making an investment decision and does not constitute a recommendation. Any opinions of the chapter authors are those of the chapter author and not necessarily those of RJFS or Raymond James. Expressions of opinion are as of the initial book publishing date and are subject to change without notice.

Raymond James Financial Services, Inc. is not responsible for the consequences of any particular transaction or investment decision based on the content of this book. All financial, retirement and estate planning should be individualized as each person's situation is unique.

This information is not intended as a solicitation or an offer to buy or sell any security referred to herein. Keep in mind that there is no assurance that our recommendations or strategies will ultimately be successful or profitable nor protect against a loss. There may also be the potential for missed growth opportunities that may occur after the sale of an investment. Recommendations, specific investments or strategies discussed may not be suitable for all investors. Past performance may not be indicative of future results. You should discuss any tax or legal matters with the appropriate professional.

Glossary

- **Assignment:** An agreement by your doctor, provider or supplier to be paid directly by Medicare, to accept the payment amount Medicare approves for the service and agrees not to bill you for any more than the Medicare deductible and coinsurance.

- **Benefit Period:** Benefit periods have nothing to do with the calendar year or coverage year. Because Part A works with inpatient hospital care, a new benefit period begins the day you enter a hospital or skilled nursing facility and ends when you have not received inpatient hospital or Medicare-covered skilled care in a skilled nursing facility for 60 days in a row. If you do require inpatient care after the 60 days has passed, a new benefit period begins. There is no limit to how many benefit periods you can have nor how long a benefit period can be.

- **Coinsurance:** This is the portion of medical expenses you are responsible for paying after your premiums and deductibles are paid for.

- **Copayment:** A payment made by the insured in addition to that made by the insurer.

- **Deductible:** The amount you must pay for your health care before Medicare begins to pay either per benefit period (for Part A) or per year (for Part B).

- **Effective Coverage Date:** The date your health insurance coverage will begin helping to pay for your medical expenses.

- **Enrollment Period:** The time period during which eligible people can sign up for different Medicare health plans. There are initial enrollment periods, general enrollment periods, open enrollment periods and special enrollment periods. (Chapter 5)

- **Formulary:** The list of drugs covered by a Part D prescription drug plan. These are different for each plan. (Chapter 2 & 14)

- **Guaranteed Access/Issue Rights:** If you enroll during certain enrollment periods, insurance companies are required by law to sell or offer you a Medigap policy. During these periods, they cannot deny you for pre-existing conditions and must offer you the best rates based on general terms – not for past or present health conditions.

- **Guaranteed Renewable:** An insurer must automatically renew your existing coverage as you are currently enrolled. The only exceptions are failing to make premium payments or having committed fraud.

- **Hospice Care:** Care designed to give supportive care to people in the final phase of a terminal illness. It focuses on comfort and quality of life, rather than finding a cure.

- **Initial Enrollment Period:** The seven-month period surrounding your 65th birthday.

- **Inpatient Care:** Medical treatment administered to a patient whose condition requires treatment in a hospital or other healthcare facility.

- **IRMAA:** Income-Related Monthly Adjustment Amounts. An adjustment (increase) charged to Medicare enrollees with higher incomes. This amount is reassessed each year.

- **Lifetime Reserve Day:** Lifetime reserve days are 60 additional days that Medicare Part A will pay for when a beneficiary is in a hospital for more than 90 days during a benefit period. As the name implies, beneficiaries are limited to a total of 60 reserve days over their lifetime. (Chapter 4 & 5)

- **Long-Term Care:** Custodial care provided in a facility or within a patient's home.

- **Medically Necessary:** Health care services or supplies needed to diagnose or treat an illness, injury, condition, disease or its symptoms that meet accepted standards of medicine.

- **Medicare-Approved Amount:** This is the amount a doctor or supplier that accepts assignment can be paid. It may be less than the actual amount a doctor or supplier charges. Medicare pays part of this amount and you are responsible for the difference.

- **Medicare Supplement Insurance:** Another name for Medigap policies.

- **Original Medicare:** Parts A & B.

- **Out-of-Network:** A doctor or network outside of a plan's contracted network of providers.

- **Outpatient Care:** Care or treatment provided that does not require an overnight stay in a hospital or medical facility.

- **Provider:** A doctor or qualified medical professional providing treatment.

- **Referral:** A written order from your primary care physician for you to see a specialist or to receive certain medical services.

- **Skilled Nursing Facility:** An in-patient rehabilitation center staffed with trained medical professionals

- **Special Enrollment Period:** The eight-month enrollment window following retirement or loss of medical coverage after age 65 (if the first month falls outside of the Initial Enrollment Period.)

- **Supplementary Medical Insurance:** Another name for Part B coverage.

- **TRICARE / TRICARE for Life:** Medical coverage provided for current and retired uniformed service members and their families.

Bibliography

Footnotes:

(1) 66% of bankruptcies tied to medical issues: https://www.cnbc.com/2019/02/11/this-is-the-real-reason-most-americans-file-for-bankruptcy.html

(2) Kaiser KFF Link: https://www.kff.org/medicare/fact-sheet/medicare-advantage/

Acknowledgments

Thanks to my mom for being editor in chief. I can assure you, dear reader, that any errors, omissions, typos or any other blemishes that remain are my own.

To my wife and family who support and encourage every crazy idea I come up with. I am more grateful for you than I could ever adequately express.

Finally, thanks to you for reading. It has been a dream of mine to write a book and am thankful you have chosen to spend your time with me. I do not take that responsibility lightly.

About the Author

Ashby Daniels is a Financial Advisor and CERTIFIED FINANCIAL PLANNER™ professional with Shorebridge Wealth Management located in Pittsburgh, PA. He works with people at or nearing retirement and assists them every step of the way at this critical juncture of their lives.

He actively writes a blog called Retirement Field Guide at https://retirementfieldguide.com/ and can be contacted via email at daniels@shorebridgewm.com.

Contact information:

Ashby Daniels, Financial Advisor

Shorebridge Wealth Management

600 Waterfront Drive, Suite 125

Pittsburgh, PA 15222

412-742-4850

Investment advisory services offered through Raymond James Financial Services Advisors, Inc. Securities offered through Raymond James Financial Services, Inc., member FINRA / SIPC.

Shorebridge Wealth Management is not a registered broker/dealer and is independent of Raymond James Financial Services, Inc.

13660446R00059